Table of Contents

Introduction

The best and most effective diet for you is one that works with your body's natural processes and systems to help you lose weight and feel the best you can in your own skin. The Alkaline Diet is believed to advantage of this and was developed to balance the pH level that naturally occurs in your body.In this book we will discuss the science and believed nutritional benefits to being on the Alkaline Diet, give you a list of alkaline friendly foods, and show you some delicious and quick smoothie recipes to help you get started.

Why Should You Go on a Diet?

How many times have you heard about someone's unsuccessful attempt at dieting? Chances are that even you failed at following a specific type of eating plan. This happens often because most people don't have a good reason to go on a diet. If your only aim is to lose weight and physically look better, it'll only be a matter of time before you get back to your unhealthy eating habits. In order to have the motivation to commit to eating only certain foods, you will have to start doing it to improve your health.The whole point of a diet is to improve the way you feel and keep you healthy. If you currently have unhealthy eating habits one of the worst things you can do is suddenly begin following an extremely strict meal plan. Completely changing when, what, and how you eat at once will make you regret it sooner rather than later and you'll likely become discouraged to make another attempt at dieting in the future. Instead, you should gradually cut out certain foods and replace them with healthy alternatives. Know that a good diet isn't supposed to be hard. In fact, it should help you feel happy and energized.

Why Choose the Alkaline Diet?

Alkaline Diet FoodsNowadays, there are a huge number of diets to choose from, so what makes this one so special? While you'll probably start losing weight as the result of an alkaline eating plan because you'll consume more fruits and veggies, the main benefit of it is that it'll lower your risk of developing serious health problems like cancer and arthritis. In case your only goal is to lose weight, we have a different list of smoothie recipes for you.

The whole idea behind the alkaline diet is to change the pH value of your body. Although there are currently no reliable studies that prove it, consuming specific foods may help make your body more alkaline. Note that when you eat unhealthy foods like refined sugar, meat, and wheat, your body will produce acidic metabolic waste when it breaks them down. It is believed that this acidic metabolic waste makes you more vulnerable to disease and illness.

If you try to Google the alkaline diet, you'll probably notice quite a few articles questioning whether it really works. It's worth noting that the claim of food affecting your blood's pH level is a myth. You can't change it with food, nor should you try doing it because your body needs to maintain a neutral pH balance. However, eating alkaline foods can have an effect on the pH levels of your urine. Although some of the science behind this diet is questionable, there is no doubt it can make you healthier and more resistant to a number of diseases. After all, you'll start eating a lot more fruits, vegetables, nuts, and seeds.

The benefits for the Alkaline Diet are purported to be many:

Healthy body weight

Increased energy

Increase in overall well being

Decrease in diseases and illnesses

Advocates suggest that this program provides all of these benefits because it offsets the human body's naturally occurring acidic pH level by balancing it with alkaline foods that have a higher pH level.

In the Alkaline Diet, the foods you eat directly alter this acidity or alkalinity in the body. When your cells extract the energy (calories) from the foods you eat, you are burning these foods in a slow way. Just like burning wood leaves ash, burning foods leaves an ashy residue. That ash can be acidic, alkaline, or neutral. That ash directly affects your body's acidity – and overall well-being.

The Alkaline Diet was popularized by Robert O. Young D.Sc., Ph.D., based on his theory that to achieve optimum health, energy, and disease-free living, the human body must consume more alkaline than acidic foods and balance the inner pH levels.

Human life needs a pH level of about 7.4 (an alkaline range between 7.3 and 7.45) to survive. Basically, when the chemistry is off, the quality of life is off, too.

With the diet, you aim to eat about 70-80% of alkaline foods. So, which foods are on the other spectrum – too acidic – and that you can't eat?

WHAT IS AN ALKALINE SMOOTHIE?

An alkaline smoothie is a smoothie that has a high pH level and shouldn't cause acid reflux or GERD symptoms. Smoothies can be loaded with acid once you add in things like berries, and juices. It's important to make sure that you're not just consuming an acidic smoothie if you easily suffer from indigestion. I definitely suffer after consuming coffee. Almond milk has an alkaline composition which helps neutralize your stomach acid, so I always have that in the house, especially for smoothies.

Why Drink Alkaline Smoothies?

We've already mentioned how important it is to gradually change your eating habits if you plan on following a new diet plan. One of the easiest ways to do this is by making an alkaline breakfast smoothie in the morning. Considering how caffeinated drinks are on the list of restricted foods in an alkaline diet, you may as well find a substitute for coffee.Of course, you can drink these smoothies during any part of the day instead of a meal of your choosing. Most people choose to prepare them in the morning because cooking a healthy breakfast can take a lot of time. On the other hand, alkaline smoothies are not only delicious and healthy, but very easy to make as well. Even if you’re not fully committed to following an alkaline diet, these are some of the healthiest smoothies you can drink, so make sure you start making them regularly.

Spinach/Kale

These two powerhouse dark green veggies are packed with health benefits. Fresh spinach is high in niacin, iron, zinc, protein, fiber, and Vitamins A, B6, C, E, and K. Kale is high in alkaline-forming minerals that include calcium and magnesium. Its very high chlorophyll content contributes to its alkaline properties, too.

Vegetables

Generally you can eat as many green as you want for the Alkaline diet. There is a whole variety of leafy greens that can rotate through in your smoothies.

Banana

Generally you want to avoid a lot of fruits which can be acid-forming. In moderation, bananas are a good fruit to put in your alkaline smoothies because they add nice flavor. Just don’t use ripe bananas which have higher levels of sugar. Bananas also contain the alkaline-forming mineral potassium.

Coconut Milk

Coconut milk is made from the alkaline-forming coconut flesh and coconut water combined. Coconut milk is nutritious; it’s rich in fiber, vitamins B1, B3, B5, B6, C, and E, and many alkaline-forming minerals such as iron, selenium, magnesium, and calcium.

Almond Milk

The many benefits and nutritious health boosts from unsweetened almond milk are also well known. Almonds are an alkalizing nut you can have on this diet. It's a dairy free, soy free, and lactose free alternative to cow's milk, which is acidic.

As you can see from a sample of ingredients above, the Alkaline Diet includes many delicious foods you can put in your smoothies. Take a handful of a dark green leafy vegetable (spinach, kale), add your fruit or fruits, and then add your additional ingredients like Greek yogurt or almond milk. Here are some high alkaline smoothie recipes to get you started (all of these recipes will work with a single-serve blender) :

ALKALINE SMOOTHIE

Ingredients

1 cup almond milk

1 cup watermelon cubed

5 strawberries frozen

1/2 small banana

1 handful spinach fresh

1 teaspoon chia seeds

1 cup ice

Instructions

Place the ingredients into the blender as listed.

Blend the smoothie until combined.

To prevent a brown smoothie, mix the greens with the banana, chia seeds, half of the ice and half of the almond milk.

Then blend the watermelon strawberries, almond milk, and ice together.

Pour the smoothies into the same glass and enjoy.

Energizing Alkaline Smoothie with Kale, Mango and Spinach

Ingredients

2 large dinosaur kale leafs

1 handful of spinach

1 banana

1/2 c frozen chopped mango

2 thumb sized knobs of ginger

1 lemon

1 c water

Instructions

Wash kale and spinach, peel lemon (leaving pith on), then toss all ingredients into blender and blend until smooth for about 1 minute.

Minty Alkaline Kiwi Green Smoothie

Ingredients

1 kiowi , sliced in half and flesh spooned out

1 green apple, peeled , peeled and sliced

1/2 English cucumber , diced (skin on)

1 cup spinach , tightly packed

Small handful fresh mint , about 10 large leaves

2 tsp pure honey

1 tsp lemon zest

juice of 1/2 lemon , medium

1 banana

1/4 cup water

1 tbsp raw coconut oil , optional

Instruction

Blitz all ingredients together in a blender for 30 - 60 seconds or until smooth and creamy. Add more honey or an extra banana for more sweetness if desired.

Alkaline Blueberry Banana

Ingredients

1 ripe banana

1/2 cup blueberries

1 teaspoon alkaline greens powder

1/2 tablespoon ground flaxseed, optional

1/2 tablespoon hemp seeds, optional

1/2 cup ice

1/2 cup milk of choice (I used soy)

1/2 cup water

Instructions

Place banana, blueberries, alkaline greens powder, flaxseed (if using), hemp seeds (if using), ice, milk, and water in a blender.

Cover and blend until ingredients are processed and smooth, about 1-2 minutes. Optional: garnish with blueberries and hemp seeds. Enjoy!

Alkaline Electric Burro Banana

INGREDIENTS

1 teaspoon of baobab powder

5 burro bananas

2 small pieces of organic lemon peel

Handful of mangoes

Handful of pumpkin seeds

A small piece of turmeric

250ml of spring water

INSTRUCTIONS

Add the following ingredients to a blending cup: burro bananas, baobab powder, lemon peels, mangoes, pumpkin seeds and turmeric.

Add 250ml of spring water to the blending cup.

Start to blend. Begin the blender on a low speed and gradually increase to full speed. This will ensure that the ingredients are well mixed together without the blades getting stuck.

Once blended, pour the smoothie into a glass and enjoy your nutritionally rich alkaline smoothie.

Enjoy.

Cucumber And Kale Smoothie

Ingredients

½ cucumber.

A handful of green curly kale.

1 tsp clear honey.

1 cup/ 250 ml/ 8.45 fl.oz coconut water.

A squeeze of lemon juice (optional, see the note).

1 tsp ginger juice from 1-inch of root ginger (optional, see the note)

Instructions

Wash and rinse the cucumber. Cut it into small pieces and place them in a blender.

Wash and rinse the Kale leaves and add them into the cucumber.

Add the rest of the ingredients into the blender.

Blend and process the cucumber mix until you get a well-mixed smoothie.

Triple Berry Smoothie

Ingredients

1 cup alkaline water

1 cup frozen blueberries

1/2 cup frozen raspberries

1/2 cup frozen blackberries

1/2 cup cooked quinoa

2 Medjool dates, halved and pitted

Instructions

Add the water, blueberries, raspberries, blackberries, quinoa, and dates into a high-speed blender. Blend on high for 60 seconds, or until it reaches a smooth consistency.

Serve immediately.

Alkaline Green Power Smoothie

INGREDIENTS

1/2 cup unsweetened rice milk

1/4 cup unsweetened dairy-free yogurt

1 cup baby kale

1 apple, core removed and diced

2–4 ice cubes

1 tablespoon coconut oil, melted

Optional: 1-2 teaspoons maple syrup and a squeeze of lemon juice, to taste

INSTRUCTIONS

1. Add all ingredients except coconut oil into the blender. Blend until smooth, adding more rice milk as needed to blend and achieve desired consistency.

2. While the blender is running, open the cap in the lid and slowly stream in your melted coconut oil. This prevents the oil from clumping. Add maple syrup and a squeeze of lemon juice to taste.

RASPBERRY SMOOTHIE

Ingredients

2 cups spinach

1 cup coconut milk

1 cup coconut water

3 cups raspberries

1 Tablespoon ground flax seed or chia seeds

1 teaspoon vanilla extract

OPTIONAL: garnish with coconut flakes, flax seed

Method

Blend spinach and liquid until smooth.

Add remaining ingredients, and blend until smooth. Garnish with coconut flakes and flax seed if you'd like, and enjoy!

PROTEIN MANGO ORANGE SMOOTHIE

Ingredients

½ cup Karuna Rejuvenate Whole Plant Juice

1 organic orange, peeled and sliced

1 tablespoon orange zest

½ cup frozen mangos

1 small baby banana or ½ large banana, very ripe

1 teaspoon fresh ginger, peeled and chopped

1 teaspoon fresh turmeric, peeled and chopped

3 tablespoons whole hemp seeds

Instructions

Add all your ingredients to a highspeed blender and blend until smooth. Serve immediately.

Smoothie will keep in the fridge for up to 24 hours and can be frozen for up to 7 days.

Alkaline Antioxidant Green Smoothie

Ingredients

A handful of Kale

A handful of Spinach

2 Broccoli heads

1 Tomato

A handful of Lettuce

1 Avocado

1 Cucumber

1/2 clove Garlic

Juice of 1/2 Lemon

A little water to the texture you like

INSTRUCTIONS

All you have to do is blend it all up! Start by blending the avocado, cucumber and lemon juice to form a mushy paste, then start adding the other ingredients.

Tropical Green Smoothie

Ingredients:

½ cup Frozen cut up banana, mango + pineapple

1 cup Unsweetened Almond Milk

1 cup Baby Spinach

1 tbsp Raw Almond Butter (I used Better Almond Butter)

1 Scoop vanilla plant based protein

1 Scoop Alkaline Greens Powder (Optional)

1 tbsp Chia Seeds or Flax

Directions:

Combine all ingredients in a blender and enjoy! Add ice if desired.

BLOOD DETOXIFYING + ALKALIZING + CANCER PREVENTING SMOOTHIE

INGREDIENTS

1 cup organic kale

2 shots organic wheatgrass

1/2 lime with pith

1 organic kiwi

1 fresh sprig of parsley

8 green organic grapes

1 Tbsp. hemp seeds or hemp powder

1 banana

INSTRUCTIONS

Blend all ingredients in a high-powered blender and serve.

GREEN GODDESS DETOX SMOOTHIE

Ingredients

2 cups baby spinach

1/4 cup kale

1 apple peeled, cored and chopped

1/2 celery stalk chopped

1/2 tablespoon ground ginger

1/4 teaspoon ground cinnamon

1/4 teaspoon turmeric

1/2 teaspoon chia seeds, flax seeds or both

1 medium carrot chopped (about 1/3 cup)

1 cup frozen mango chunks

1/2 cup frozen pineapple chunks

1/2 lemon peeled and chopped

1 cup water or more depending on the consistency you prefer (I use water kefir but feel free to use what you have - coconut water would be great too)

Instructions

Place all the ingredients in your high-performance blender (I used the Blendtec) in the order as they appear.

Blend on high until completely smooth or until desired consistency is reached. Feel free to add more or less water depending on the consistency you prefer.

Spinach & Strawberry Super Smoothie

Ingredient

2 cups spinach

½ cup strawberries

1 lime

1 banana

1 cup coconut water

1 tbsp hemp seeds

1 scoop of alkalizer & detoxifier powder

Instructions

Simply put all of the ingredients in a blender and blend them until smooth. Note that the banana can be either fresh or frozen. Don’t place the whole lime in the blender but instead squeeze the juice out of it. Although the smoothie will likely already be sweet, you can add some stevia to sweeten it.

Kiwi & Cucumber Smoothie

Ingredients

1 kiwi fruit

¼ cucumbers

½ bananas

1 handful of spinach

3-4 almonds

¼ cup coconut milk

Instructions

Combine all of these ingredients and blend them. In case you want to make this alkalizing smoothie more refreshing, add a few ice cubes in the blender.

Alkaline Breakfast Smoothie

Ingredients

1 cup kale

1 banana

½ cup strawberries

1 cup orange juice

¼ cup raspberries

Instructions

The raspberries, strawberries, and banana can all be either fresh or frozen. Mix the ingredients in a blender and add a few ice cubes to make it more refreshing.

ALKALINE CHERRY SMOOTHIE

INGREDIENTS

1-½ cup almond milk

1 cup fresh cherries, seeded

1 cup fresh kale, stems removed

1 kiwi peeled

2 tbsp raw cashews

½ fresh beet, chopped

INSTRUCTIONS

Add all ingredients to high speed blender.

Blend until smooth.

Raw Vegan Alkaline Green Smoothie

INGREDIENTS

4 cups firmly packed organic baby spinach leaves

1 cup filtered water

1 medium avocado

juice of 1 red ruby grapefruit

1 English cucumber chopped

1 or 2 cups of ice cubes depending on preference

1 inch piece of raw creamed coconut

3 Tbsp coconut crystals or a few drops of stevia depending on your preference.

DIRECTIONS

Throw all of your ingredients in your blender and puree until smooth and creamy.

Adjust sweetener to taste and devour.

ALKALINE BROCCOLI-BLUEBERRY-SPINACH SMOOTHIE

Ingredients

5 broccoli florets

2 bananas

50g spinach

1/2 cup frozen blueberries

1/2 orange

1/4 cup almond milk

1 tbsp almond meal

1 tbsp almond date paste (almond meal+dates, blended)

Instructions

Throw everything into the blender and blast on high.

Fruit Infused Sea Moss Gel Recipe

Ingredients

0.5 oz (about 14 grams when weighed) Raw Unsoaked Sea Moss, or 5.5 oz soaked sea moss (~156 grams)

1 cup Fresh or Frozen Fruit, cut into cubes

5 Medjool Dates, pitted and soaked for at least 30 minutes

1 cup Alkaline Water

Instructions

Place the dried sea moss in a large bowl, cover it with water, and massage the sea moss. Be sure to remove any visible dirt and debris. Drain and repeat this step once more

Place the sea moss in a large bowl and cover it with filtered or spring water. (do not use tap water) Make sure all the parts of the sea moss are covered. Allow the sea moss to soak for 12-24 hours. (at room temperature)

Add the soaked sea moss to the blender, along with the dates, fruit, and water.

Blend until it is smooth, about 1-3 minutes. Transfer the Sea Moss into an airtight container/mason jar, and refrigerate. The sea moss gel will thicken in the fridge \after 2 hours.

Transfer the Sea Moss into an airtight mason jar. Store in the refrigerator for 3-4 weeks or in the freezer for up to 3 months.

Avocado Lime Breakfast Smoothie

Ingredients:

3/4 cup (75g) cucumber with peel

3 cups (85g) baby spinach

2 cups (200g) frozen Broccoli

1/2 medium (75g) avocado

1/2 cup (115g) of organic silken tofu

1 large lime or 2 small limes, peeled

1/4 tsp. stevia extract

1/2 cup ice

1/2 cup unsweetened organic plant-based milk (I Used almond)

Directions:

Add Ingredients into a powerful high-speed blender I recommend this one ,and blend until smooth and creamy.

Serve into a bowl and enjoy!

Baby Spinach, Blueberry and Wheatgrass Smoothie

Ingredients

1 medium apple

1 cup baby spinach

1 medium banana

1 cup blueberries

1 tsp wheat grass powder

Directions

Blend all the ingredients together with as much water and ice as you like and serve.

Enjoy 1-2 tablespoons a day on its own or in smoothies, drinks and tea.

My Morning Alkaline Juice

Ingredients

2 large carrots

3 cucumbers

2 celery stalks

3 apples

1 cup spinach

Directions

Carefully wash all the ingredients.

Peel the carrots.

Cut vegetables into chunks that would fit into your juicer.

When cutting the apples, remove their core.

Juice the apples and vegetables alternating the ingredients for better results.

Matcha and alkalising greens smoothie

Ingredients

½ cup

Cucumbers, chopped

2 Tbsp

Avocados

1 handful

Fresh mint

1 large handful

Spinach, or other leafy greens like kale (Main)

¾ tsp

Matcha (green tea) powder, see buying tips below (Main)

⅓ cup

Coconut water, or regular filtered water (Main)

⅓ cup

Coconut milk, See link above for an easy recipe to make your own (Main)

½ cup

Ice

Directions

Place everything in a high speed blender and blend until completely smooth.

Pour into a tall glass and enjoy.

DETOXIFY WEIGHT LOSS JUICE

Ingredients:

5 Stalk – Fresh Organic Celery, washed and diced

1 medium size – Bottle Gourd, peeled, washed and diced

¼ cup – Fresh Coriander Leaves with Stalk (Optional)

4 Sprigs – Curry Leaves or Sweet Neem Leaves, washed(Optional)

Instructions

Using a cold-press Omega juicer (Or any slow-juicer) and start adding & juicing the above ingredients

Alternatively, add above ingredients to a Vitamix blender with ¼ cup of water and blend to a smooth puree, & strain it.

Enjoy this light refreshing green juice.

C Punch Smoothie

Ingredients

1 cup water

1 banana

1 orange

1/2 cup fresh mango

1 cup packed spinach

1 cup ice

Instructions

Add ingredients to the jar and secure lid. Blend until smooth.

For Blendtec: Press the SMOOTHIE Button

For Vitamix: Select VARIABLE, speed #1. Turn on machine and quickly increase speed to #10; then to HIGH. Run for 45 seconds or until smooth.

Transfer to a glass and serve immediately.

To store, pour into a glass container and keep in the fridge for 1-2 days. Alternatively, pour into a plastic container and freeze for up to 1 month.

All done! Enjoy!! Now take a photo, rate it, and share your accomplishments!

Raw Green Savory Breakfast Smoothie

INGREDIENTS

1 tomato (chopped)

½ english cucumber (peeled and chopped)

1 avocado

¼ bunch cilantro (or parsley if preferred)

1 lime (peeled and chopped)

¼ medium onion (chopped)

½ head Romaine lettuce–or of your choice (chopped)

1 teaspoon sea salt

2 tablespoons omega-rich oil (we used a blend of flax, sesame, and sunflower oil)

INSTRUCTIONS

Place all ingredients in blender and blend until chunky or smooth, depending upon your preference.

Enjoy!

Anti-Bloat Smoothie

Ingredients

1/2 c alkaline water

1 banana, peeled and frozen overnight

1 large cucumber, sliced

1 inch piece of fresh ginger, peeled and sliced

handful of ice

Instructions

Add all of the ingredients to a blender and pulse until you get a smoothie consistency.

If you feel extra hardcore, stir in 1 tablespoon of raw apple cider vinegar into your smoothie.

WHOLE FOODS IRON RICH SMOOTHIE

Ingredients

1/2 cup beet cut into small cubes

1 cup frozen raspberries

1 medium orange peeled

1 apple chopped

1 heaping tablespoon of hemp seeds

1/2 cup alkaline water

Instructions

Put all ingredients into a high powered blender like a Vitamix and blend until smooth.

REFRESHING GREEN SMOOTHIE

INGREDIENTS

250g spinach

1 lime

1 banana

2 kiwi

INSTRUCTIONS

Peel the lime and blend everything together to make a healthy green smoothie.

Consume the green smoothie as soon as it's made as it will begin to oxidise.

Chew your green smoothie to make it digested easier. Swallow just as it warms to body temp.

Alkaline Diet Green Juice

Ingredients

2 Organic Carrots, washed and peeled

1 Organic Cucumber

1/4 Organic Head Green Cabbage

1 cup Organic Spinach

1/2 Organic Lime

Directions

Wash and chop ingredients to fit into juicer.

Process ingredients in order through juicer.

Drink now or store in refrigerator for up to 48 hours.

Morning Pineapple Ginger Green Smoothie

INGREDIENTS

2 cups Filtered Water

4 cups Spinach

1 Frozen Banana

2 cups Frozen Pineapple

1 Tbs Fresh Ginger

½ Lemon freshly squeezed

INSTRUCTIONS

Add water and greens to the blender and blender until smooth.

Add banana, pineapple, ginger, and lemon juice. Blend thoroughly.

Best served immediately after blending!

Anti-Cancer Green Smoothie Recipe

ingredients

1/4 cup hemp seeds

2 cups carrot juice

1 cup water

1 ripe banana, frozen

1 cup frozen strawberries

1 cup frozen broccoli florets

2 cups fresh or lightly steamed baby kale or baby spinach

5 fresh mint leaves

2 tablespoons cocoa powder

1/2 lime or lemon, juiced

instructions

Combine the hemp seeds, carrot juice, and water in the base of a high-speed blender like a Vitamix or Blendtec.

Next, add the frozen banana, frozen strawberries, frozen broccoli florets, greens, mint, cocoa powder, and lemon or lime juice.

Place the lid on the blender and blend until smooth, about 45 seconds.

Serve immediately.

Clear Skin Diet Smoothie

INGREDIENTS

1 1/2 cups fresh spinach

1 cup coconut water, unsweetened

1 cup pineapple, frozen

1/4 avocado

1 Protein Smoothie Boost, optional

INSTRUCTIONS

Blend spinach and coconut water until smooth.

Add remaining ingredients, and blend until smooth.

Creamy Avocado Banana Green Smoothie

Ingredients

SMOOTHIE

1 large frozen banana (ripe // peeled // sliced)

1/4 – 1/2 medium ripe avocado (more avocado = creamier, thicker smoothie)

1 scoop plain or vanilla protein powder (see my Protein Powder Guide here)

1 large handful greens of choice (spinach, kale, rainbow chard // I like mine frozen)

3/4 – 1 cup unsweetened plain almond milk (or any dairy-free milk)

ADD-INS optional

1 Tbsp seed of choice (hemp, flax, sesame, sunflower, chia, etc.)

1/2 tsp adaptogen of choice (maca, ashwagandha, etc.)

1/2 cup sliced frozen (or fresh) cucumber or berries (organic when possible)

Instructions

To a high-speed blender, add frozen banana, avocado, protein powder of choice, greens, and dairy-free milk. At this time, add any desired add-ins, such as adaptogens, seeds, or additional fruits and vegetables (such as berries or cucumbers).

Blend on high until creamy and smooth, scraping down sides as needed. If smoothie is too thick, add more dairy-free milk to thin. If too thin, add more frozen banana or avocado.

Taste and adjust flavor as needed, adding more banana for sweetness, avocado for creaminess, or greens for vibrant green color. Protein powder can also be used to add more sweetness (depending on brand / flavor).

Divide between serving glasses and enjoy! Best when fresh, though leftovers will keep covered in the refrigerator up to 24 hours or in the freezer up to 2 weeks.

conclusion

While there currently isn't a lot of medical research that has been done on the Alkaline Diet, the diet's emphasis on eating more vegetables and fruits and removing processed foods are good guidelines to follow.The hardest aspect of this diet is following it due to the many food restrictions, but adding any of these alkaline-friendly smoothies to your diet is a good way to start.

www.ingramcontent.com/pod-product-compliance
Ingram Content Group UK Ltd.
Pitfield, Milton Keynes, MK11 3LW, UK
UKHW021656190726
13853UKWH00001B/297